ANIMAL AND VEGETABLE PARASITES OF THE HUMAN SKIN AND HAIR;

T0025885

ANIMAL AND VEGETABLE PARASITES OF THE HUMAN SKIN AND HAIR;

Benjamin Joy Jeffries

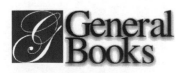

www.General-Books.net

Publication Data:

Title: Animal and Vegetable Parasites of the Human Skin and Hair
Author: Benjamin Joy Jeffries
General Books publication date: 2009
Original publication date: 1872
Original Publisher: A. Moore
Subjects: Medical parasitology
Medical / Parasitology
Science / Life Sciences / Biology / Microbiology
Science / Life Sciences / Zoology / General

1

SECTION 1

ANIMAL PARASITES
   OF THE HUMAN SKIN.
   CHAPTER I.

Man's cutaneous envelope, like the integument of the lower animals, is subject to be temporarily visited by parasites, or perhaps become a permanent abode for them. However unpleasant this idea may seem, only too many of the human family in the most civilized countries are annoyed or rendered miserable by the presence of the animal parasites. Amongst the poor and dirty, the unfortunate children suffer a great deal from them, and we have seen serious trouble arise from their ravages. But all classes of the community are liable to be infested by them, – the wealthiest and the cleanest. Among the lower classes, prejudice, ignorance, and even superstition, help to favor the production and continued existence of these parasites ; and in the upper

classes a lack of knowledge of their nature, and the means to avoid or get rid of them. The mental agony of a young lady on finding her auburn tresses the home of the only too common insect, can only be appreciated by those who have realized it. We have known the most refined to suffer thus for months, merely from shame to apply to a physician, or ignorance of the very simple means necessary to be freed from what is naturally regarded as so loathsome. Where soap and water are attainable, man can keep his body clear of these animals. If every teacher in the public schools could be authorized to send a child so infested home, and at the same time knew enough to direct the mother or family what to do to relieve the child of its trouble, it would at least be a comfort to those physicians who, in attendance at the great charitable institutions, come necessarily in immediate contact with the thousands of poor people and their little ones, whom sickness and misery are constantly sending there. The animal parasites are the pest of the public schools. Neglect and ignorance alone foster their presence. By explaining the natural history, the habits, habitats, methods of propagating, and

means of getting rid of these animals, we hope to be able to assist our readers in keeping a *mens sana in corpore sano,* – a sound mind in a healthy and *cleanly* body.

The animal parasites of the human skin may be divided into two classes : those which live *on* the skin, and those whiph live *in* the skin. We will commence our study with those of the first class, namely, the *pediculi,* of which there are three kinds, – the *head-louse,* the *crab-louse',* and the *body-louse.* The first of these is met with only on the hair of the head; it is entirely confined to the scalp, and never attacks the other hairy parts of the body. It is unfortunately too familiar an object to require any special delineation of it to be given here. The color varies, livid or pale gray, and is said to change according to the hair. The male insects are fewer in number than the females; the latter are also much larger. They have three pairs of legs, and all the feet are similar. The last tarsal joint has a large claw on its outside, and on its inside two straight, thick, horny stumps, and a large bristle. A microscope of moderate magnifying power will show this structure of the animal.

When the eggs are laid, they stick firmly to the human hair, and are called *nits.* This we will more particularly explain further on. In six days the young escape from the egg, and are ready to lay eggs at the age of eighteen days. A female lays some fifty eggs in all. We thus see why such enormous quantities of the animals are often seen, and how they propagate with such astonishing rapidity.

It is easy enough to tell when a person is infested with these vermin, because the animals creep about upon the head, and their eggs are large enough to betray themselves to the naked eye, especially on dark hair. As the insect can run about, the eggs will be found strung along the whole length of the hair.

We said this kind inhabits only the scalp, where, by their creeping about, but more especially by their biting the skin, in pursuit of nourishment, they cause intense and constant itching, and hence intense and constant scratching on the part of the person infested. We all know how tender the scalp is made by hard brushing, combing, or violent shampooing, and can therefore readily understand that the constant digging the finger-nailsinto the skin of the head to allay the itching, will finally cause inflammation of the cutaneous surface. An artificial *eczema,* as dermatologists call it, is produced, and this all the more in those persons, children for instance, who are predisposed to eczematous eruptions. This inflammation causes a fluid to exude from the skin, which, with the blood coming from where the cuticle has been deeply torn by the nails, dries up and forms crusts and scales, mixed also with the natural fatty secretion of the scalp, from the sebaceous follicles. Hence the loathsome appearance which such a head presents. Moreover, the greater the amount of exuded fluid, the greater amount of food for these vermin, and the more rapid their growth and multiplication. Thus we see that the irritation of the lice caused itching; this led to the scratching, which, continued for a length of time, produced an artificial eczema, or inflammation of the skin. The exuded fluid of eczema is food for the *pediculi,* under the crusts and scales the animals can hide ; the matted hair affords better opportunity for the eggs or *nits* to hatch, and so a person who has eczema of the head offers a much better field for the cultivation and propagation of these vermin.

Now dirt and poverty predispose to eczematous eruptions; and those with such disease are, in these circumstances of life, more liable to come in contact with others infested with *pediculi,* and thus the animals are transferred from one person to another. We all know how quickly one infested head in a school, or public institution, affects the other children, even when considerable care and cleanliness are exercised. But these insects never come except from contagion. The vermin crawl from one person to another. The eggs or nits are not transferred, for these adhere tenaciously to the hairs where they are deposited by the female insect. All stories of the *spontaneous generation* of these or any other vermin are simply ridiculous, and arise from ignorance, and the lack of accurate and truthful observation. Care and cleanliness are necessary on the part of all who are forced to come in immediate contact with the dirty and squalid. Some sympathy, we hold, should be felt by the community for physicians who are obliged to do this, as it is quite as disagreeable for them as for others. Moreover, to say they are *used to it* is no argument, since the *getting*
used to it involves what others never have to undergo.

Probably the human race all over the world are infested more or less *withpediculi.* It is even doubtful whether there are different species of this insect, or *pediculus capitis.* One observer thought he found a particular species on African negroes. Lice are described as being rare among the Brazilian Indians, and among the Indians of Magda- lena, in Columbia; but travellers have found them among the New Hollanders, and the Asiatic and American Indians. . Their dried brood has been found in the hair of the Peruvian mummies. At one time it was asserted that there was a particular *pediculus tabescentium,* or louse of the consumptive, and good people rather preferred to be supposed to have them than the common head- louse, *which, however, they were.*

The next animal parasite of the human skin, whose natural history we will study, is *the pediculus pubis,* or crab-louse, which resembles the *pediculus capitis,* but is shorter and broader. It does not run about on the surface, but grasps the hair close down to the skin with its fore-legs, which are provided with strong crab-like claws. The animal holds on so tight, that it will be crushed before it relaxes the grasp of the hair; it deposits its eggs, the nits, on the hair, just as the *pediculus capitis* does; but as it cannot run about, these are always placed on the hair close to the skin, and hence often *overlooked.* To this we shall recur again, when speaking of the treatment of these vermin. This animal lives on all the haired portions of the body *except the scalp,* which is the domain of the *pediculus capitis.* They never interfere with each other. When both are present on the same person, the head-louse will be found on the hair of the head, down, for instance, to the whisker, and never below; whilst the orab-louse infests the whiskers up to the scalp, which he never occupies; he does, however, take possession of the eyebrows and eyelashes. Why this is, is not yet known. The insect is transferred from one individual to another by contact, and by the agency of clothes, linen, and beds. It is said to be most abundant in southern climates.

This *pediculus* lives on human blood, and, in obtaining it from the skin by biting deeply and firmly, it causes often considerable irritation, varying, of course, with the cutaneous sensibilityof the person affected. This itching calls for scratching, -which finally produces a papular, or eczematous eruption, the seat of which, however, points towards the cause, and a careful examination will detect the *pediadi* on the hair close to the skin, and the nits also near by. As these parasites do not cause so much irritation as the *pediculi capitis,* and infesting portions of the body covered by the clothing, they often remain unobserved, frequently living and thriving on an individual for an indefinite period, especially among those whose change of raiment or ablutions occur about as often as the equinoxes, but not with the same regularity. The ravages of the head-louse, and the ravages of the finger-nails and comb to allay the itching of the scalp, often produce, as we said, an artificial *eczema,* or inflammation of the skin, which, when long continued and excessive, may finally cause the glands in the neighborhood to swell up or break down into abscesses on the neck, for instance, or behind the ears. This rarely occurs with the *pediculus pubis;* yet in a person predisposed to glandular swellings, the glands in the groin may swell up from long-continued scratching, and consequent eczematous eruptions, from this insect. But pustules are not so readily caused on the other haired portion of the body as on the scalp; moreover, the head being uncovered, is readily scratched when infested by vermin, and the deep digging of the finger-nails is more irritating than the rubbing of the clothes.

The third and last pediculus to be described is the *pediculus vestimenti,* clothes-louse, or body- louse. It is similar to the *pediculus capitis* in external form, only larger, the principal distinction being the size. It is whitish in color, and from one-twelfth to one-sixth of an inch in length. There are three legs on each side, having four joints, and terminating in claws. The habitat, or place of living of the insect, is the clothes, in the folds and seams of which the eggs are deposited, appearing as little yellowish-white shining dots. It feeds by biting the skin – principally those parts nearest its haunt: namely, where the clothes come in most immediate and constant contact with the cutaneous surface. Hence its ravages are seen on the neck, back, and shoulders, around the waist, and wherever bands or straps give a resting-place for the insects, an opportunity for the eggs t& hatch undisturbed, and by lack of change of ap-parel, a constant field of food. But though the skin is mostly affected at these parts, any portion of it which is covered may show signs of the vermin, since the patient will not only scratch where the insect bites, but any part of the cutaneous surface ; it being a well-known fact, that to allay the sensation of itching it is not necessary to scratch exactly where the source of irritation exists.

Since the insect lives in the recesses of the clothes, and sallies forth from there to prey upon the skin for existence, a person so affected is quite free of vermin when naked, a few adhering to the skin, whilst the clothing removed may be a living mass of them. It is the constant wearing of the same clothing, therefore, which affords a permanent home for these insects. According to the numbers present, and the cuta-neous sensibility of the individual infested, will be the amount of irritation produced, and the consequent amount of scratching. At first the slight itching occasions only streaks of white or red from the marks of the finger-nails, but afterwards excoriations are seen from the further injury of the skin. These excoriations will have little drops of dried blood, the skin becomes quite red, and, as with the other forms of pediculi, exhibits the scabs described – papules, vesicles, and pustules. When the insects have preyed upon the individual. for a long time, the continued irritation causes continued congestion and infiltration, increasing the deposit of pigment in the skin, which finally becomes rougher, darker, and thicker than natural – sometimes absolutely as black as the negro's.

The presence of these vermin, as with the other kinds, cause, *from the scratching,* artificial ecze- inatous eruptions, and in general call forth, on the cutaneous surface, any disease of this tissue to which the individual so affected is liable, or predisposed to. The enormous numbers of these vermin which have at times been seen, and their apparently rapid production, has given rise to the idea that they were also generated spontaneously. But this, as we said above, is owing to incorrect observation and erroneous deduction. The *pediculi vestimenti,* like the other pediculi, thrive best when let alone, and where morbid cutaneous secretions attract them. They may be always detected on the clothing, if not on the body. The

general domain of their ravages tells the dermatologist what insect he has to deal with.

In the old days of superstition and credulity, the death of any person specially noted in history was very apt to be attributed by those succeeding them, or those who wrote their history, to the ravages of these several forms of lice, especially this last – the clothes-louse. For instance, Aristotle relates that the poet Alcmanes, and the Syrian Pherecydes, died of *phihiriasis;* i. e., of insects living on the body. Other more recent authors report the same of Herod, Sylla, even Plato, Philip the Second, and so on. However, nowadays, we understand that a person lying in bed sick, unable to move, uncleansed and neglected from superstition or otherwise, will soon attract, from those coming in contact with them, the parasites that the want of bodily ablution, and ignorance of a former age, allowed to accumulate till death might be readily attributed to them. In a civilized country, where soap and water, and medicines which kill these vermin, can be obtained, . there is no longer reason or excuse for their presence, as we shall next see.

CHAPTER II.

We have given a sketch of the habits, habitats, and appearances of the three animal parasites of the human skin which live upon it, of the family of pediculi. We also spoke of the effect upon the cutaneous surface of their seeking nourishment in the skin, the result of the intense itching caused thereby, and the consequences of the irritation from the person's endeavors to allay this. In this chapter we will endeavor to explain how and where these insects deposit their eggs, in what way they can be destroyed as well as the animals themselves, and thus enable those annoyed and chagrined by their presence to rid themselves of them and their effects.

The head-louse and the crab-louse lay their eggs on the hairs, to which they are very firmly fastened, so that endeavoring to remove them will sometimes even pull out the hair itself. They are called nits, and are strung along on the hairs like beads. The pedieulns of the head, as it can runabout, lays its eggs more scattered on the hair than the pediculus pubis, which can only move by grasping the hair with its crab-like claws, and thus pull itself from one to another; hence it lays its eggs close down to the skin on the hair, and where there are many these are strung close to each other, consequently often overlooked, even when somewhat carefully sought for. The eggs of these two insects are very much alike, and attached to the hair in the same method, so that a single description will answer for both. A proper knowledge of them is so essential to understanding the methods of destroying them, that we shall give a somewhat minute description in explanation of the figures here given. The eggs, as seen, are pear- shaped. The posterior end is pointed, the anterior truncate, and furnished with a flattened round

Fig. 1.

cover. *Fig.* 1 represents the ordinary appearance of the egg when seen with a magnifying power of about eighty diameters. We here see how the egg is fastened to the hair, and why they stick so firmly, being cemented as it were with a strongly

Fig. 2.

glutinous substance. *Fig.* 2 shows the egg when rendered transparent in the glycerine, and examined with a magnifying power of one hundred and thirty under the microscope. The broad end of the egg has a lip, to which is attached a conical lid, studded with little nodular processes. This lid falls off when the animal is ready to come out of the shell. We see such a one at the side of thehair which has come off from the egg in which the insect is curled up. In the other egg on the hair the pediculus is seen in the process of development. We now know what a nit is, and how the insect escapes from this egg. The shell is quite hard, even with difficulty broken between the finger-nails. It entirely escapes long-continued and hard combing, and is not destroyed by ordinary washing with soap and water, or shampooing. This is a point people generally are quite ignorant of, but to be especially remembered.

The other kind of pediculus which lives secreted in the folds and seams of the clothes, lays its eggs there. They are seen as minute, round, yellowish-white dots, quite different from the eggs of the other pediculi, and never found sticking to the hairs.

All these insects are regarded as loathsome, and yet every human being, from the highest to the lowest, is liable to become infested with them, for all classes of the community come in greater or less contact with each other; and it is by contact, or by clothing, or utensils, that the animals are passed from one to another. We cannot easily avoid them, but we can always readily get rid ofthem and their effect on the skin, provided they have not continued their ravages too long, for their careful treatment by those experienced in cutaneous diseases is sometimes requisite to relieve the patient of their trouble. We mean that severe and persistent inflammation of the skin is often caused by the presence, and consequent irritation, of these animals we have described, calling for the best efforts of those who have made diseases of the skin a special study, in order to subdue it.

The treatment *ofpkthiriasis,* or the presence of lice, is quite simple, if three things are borne in mind, namely: that we must kill the live insects, destroy the eggs, and care for the condition of the skin left afterwards. No w there are a number of substances of the mineral and vegetable world, which are quite deadly to these animals when brought in contact with them, such as sulphur, mercury, seeds of stavesacre, of sabadilla; the root of pyrethrum or pellitory, many of the essential oils, and alcohol. All the patent medicines and other advertised nostrums warranted to destroy these vermin contain some of these substances; but as manyof such medicines are irritating to the skin, their indiscriminate use is likely to do much harm. Sulphur can be used as vapor baths or fumigations, but equally as well in the common sulphur

ointment of the Pharmacopoeia. Its smell prevents its use by those who object to it, and other things do equally well. Mercury can be used as the common mercurial ointment, or two or three grains of the bichloride of mercury can be dissolved in an ounce of water, and a few drops of alcohol added, to assist solution. When applied to the skin in this way the danger of salivation amounts to nothing. Seeds of stavesacre can be used as ointment, one part to four of lard, or an infusion of them in vinegar. Sabadilla seeds can . be used as a powder when ground up, or as an ointment, one part to eight of lard. A few drops of the essential oils, as oil of cinnamon or rosemary added to these ointments, disguise or improve the odor. The root of the pyrethrum or pellitory is generally used in powder. Some of the strong essential oils are also serviceable.

We thus see that there are a variety of substances we can employ, some one of which is always within every one's reach. To get rid ofthese insects on the head, we must remember that although the fine tooth-comb, steadily used, will, when the hairs are not matted and there is no s%- cretiou, remove all the live animals, yet it will not destroy the nits or eggs, or break them away from their attachment to the hairs. These eggs can only be broken down by *repeated washing with alcohol* or *weak vinegar,* or the strongest soft soap, such as the German Schmierseife, or smearing soap. The cure is not complete till the hairs are free from them. When there is no objection, as in children, it is better to cut the hair short, as thereby we get rid of large numbers of nits, and can bring whatever we use in more immediate contact with the animals we desire to destroy. When the hair is matted together by secretions, and the skin inflamed, it is absolutely necessary to cut the hair short, and use steady cleansing with soap and warm water, otherwise the animals continue to propagate under the products of the inflammation, and multiply innumerably.

It is not necessary to sacrifice the hair in women. Combing, washing, and the application of some of the above remedies are quite effectual. When there is severe inflammation and much eruption onthe head, especially of children, it will be safer to consult some physician who pays especial attention to diseases of the skin; remember, however, to avoid all who advertise in any form whatever, by newspapers, handbills, pamphlets or almanacs, and equally avoid patent medicines and quack nostrums. These, unfortunately, only too often succeed in fleecing the ignorant and credulous, because the general practitioner disregards or treats but lightly what in reality needs knowledge, thought and care.

We have explained that the *pediculus pubis,* or crab-louse, lived on all the haired portions of the body *except the scalp,* which territory he always leaves intact for his cousin the *pediculus capitis.* This insect, it must again be remembered, cannot run about, but holds on to the hair close to the skin. Combing and rubbing will not dislodge it, but it is readily, like the pediculus capitis, killed by some of the substances mentioned. A powder called Capuchin powder is used in Europe, to destroy both these species of vermin. It is composed of equal parts of seeds of stavesacre, cocculus and sabadilla. To effect a cure, all parts of the body infested, or likely to be, must be thoroughlyrubbed. Some of the ointments, though not so cleanly to apply, are more effectual than the powders in destroying this insect; and washing them off with strong soap, and hard rubbing, breaks down the egg-shells, and prevents the young from hatching. Thoroughness and care are the secret of success. Any portion of the haired portion of the body neglected, may be the seat of continued contagion. The eyelashes even do not escape, and the figures we have given are drawn from the eggs of the pediculus pubis, found on the. lashes. We can understand now how it is that some tribes of men whose habits are particularly uncleanly, still manage to be comparatively free of these vermin. It is because they use strong-smelling fats and ointments for smearing the surface of the body, and rubbing into the hair in their manner of dressing it. Perhaps the necessity of some defence for the body, so much exposed in hot climates from the attacks of insects, originated the use of many ointments among savage tribes, especially those living in the tropics. In speaking of the *pediculus vestimenti,* or clothes-louse, we said, when the person infested had removed his clothes, he had removed the

insects, except any that might be then biting the skin; so that to get rid of these vermin, clean clothes and a thorough ablution is all that is necessary. After they have lived and multiplied on the individual indefinitely, as is often the case amongst the lowest classes in civilized countries, and among dirty semi-barbarous people who live in climates requiring constant clothing, then the products of the inflammation of the skin may conceal some of these insects and their eggs, render- ing an application to the skin of one of the remedies above mentioned necessary. Boiling clothes that can be washed, effectually destroys both eggs and insects. A heat of 150 degrees Fahrenheit applied to clothes that would be spoiled by boiling, will also destroy all the animals and their eggs concealed in the folds and seams. In some parts of the world the common people bury infested clothing in hay for several weeks; in this way the insects are killed, and the eggs prevented hatching. Strewing clothing with some of the powders we have mentioned above, also suflices to disinfect it, without hurting the cloth in any way. But the treatment of the clothing, like the

treatment of the skin, must be thoroughly attended to.

Of the million and a half of men who composed the Northern and Southern armies during the rebellion, we doubt if many score escaped being infested by these parasites. We should not like to say what proportion of the thousands of recruits who passed through our examination, had to be made clean before becoming soldiers. We have known of officers being furloughed from the field to return home, and once more get free of their travelling companions in the shape of vermin. Had every army surgeon, North and South, been quite familiar with the habits and habitats of these insects, much suffering might have been saved. Those who did understand the proper and efficient methods of prevention and treatment, often labored strenuously for the personal cleanliness of their command. Of course all effort failed when the accidents or necessities of war prevented for weeks, or months, perhaps, change of clothing, requisite ablutions, and the wasning of under-garments. The horrors of the Southern prisons were rendered still worse by the loathsome presence of vermin, which the inmates fruitlessly got rid of, as contagion soon caused them to become as infested as before. There was, however, great ignorance as well as great neglect. Even in times of peace, the surgical staff of our prisons, institutions of correction, school-ships, asylums, children's homes, etc., know only too well how hard it is to enforce a personal cleanliness, which shall prevent the presence of contagious vermin. With great armies in the field it is impossible; but not necessary with these in times of peace.

We do not propose to speak here of the various insects which attack man by stinging, or those which draw blood from the skin for food, as they cannot be strictly called parasites. We mean of the former class, scorpions, ants, spiders, etc., and of the latter class, bed-bugs, fleas, mosquitoes, gnats, many species of flies, etc.

We will, therefore, now pass to the consideration of some of the animal parasites which live in the skin, or which may, under certain circumstances, deposit their eggs there. The great blue-bottle fly, *musca vomitoria,* lays its eggs in the orifices of the human body, or in wounds and ulcers. The removal of their larvae is a matter of care and importance. So also with the common flesh-fly, *musca carnaria.* They thus add greatly to the misery of certain endemic diseases, as the affections of the eye in Egypt. The housefly may also deposit its eggs, and its larvae be found in wounds, and the orifices of the body. The eggs and larvse of the bot-flies may live oh the skin, and there form boils. In South America this parasite is reported as by no means rare upon man. Von Humboldt called it *oestrus hu- manus.* It is not yet, however, settled whether this is different from the bot of the horse, sheep, ox, stag, and other bot-flies. Fluctuation will be sought for in vain in the tumors produced by them, but an orifice will be found in the swelling, from which a little moisture constantly oozes, and through which the hinder part of the *oestrus* is kept in communication with the air. The prognosis is favorable, and immediate cure is only possible by incision, and the removal of the *oestrus.*

The Medina-worm, or Guinea hair-worm, *fila- ria medinencis,* is an inhabitant of another portion of the world, and need not, therefore, be discussed here. On the other hand, we must take some notice of the sand-flea, *pulex penetrans,* sinceit occurs in South America, and where our countrymen may more often come in contact with it. It is smaller than the common flea, and has a proboscis as long as the body. The male insect does not penetrate the skin. This is done by the female, which swells up extraordinarily after it has burrowed under the skin of men and auimals. Von Humboldt thought it attacked only Europeans, and not the aborigines. It is described as an animal so small that it can only be seen by sharp eyes, with a good light, for which reason the seeking for the flea, after its immigration, is generally left to children. It perforates the skin down to the flesh, and, concealed in its little canal, swells up into a white, globular vesicle, which, in a few days, may become as large as a pea, the pain constantly increasing; this is the abdomen of the female filled with eggs, or, more correctly, with larvae. Neglect of the disorder, or careless rupture of the vesicle, that is, the abdomen, by which the young are scattered in the wound, where they then mine frqsh passages, leads to bad sores, to inflammation of the glands of the groin, to mortification, and, in consequence, to amputation or mutilation of the limbs, or even to death. The toes are especially attacked by the flea, although other parts of the body are also visited. Persons who are staying in the places where the flea is common, must have their feet examined every two or three days. When the animal has once made an entrance, the orifice of the canal, which is marked by a red point, may be sought, the passage widened by a needle, and the flea drawn out, but without tearing it. With fresh punctures it is best to wait a day, until the occurrence of the white vesicle, that is to say, the swelling of the abdomen with the brood, allows the animal to be more readily detected. The cavity remaining after extraction, is treated like a simple wound. In Brazil they fill it with oil, snuff, or ashes.

There are two animals remaining for us to describe, inhabitants of the human skin. One is the *acarus scabiei,* or *sarcoptes hominis,* the itch insect, which causes no end of trouble in and on the skin. The other, and perfectly harmless parasite, of mau's cutaneous envelope, is the *acarus folliculorum,* or pimple mite, of which *Fig.* 3 is a representation. This is a very enlarged view of the animal, since its true length is from onehundredth to one-fiftieth of an inch in length. Our figure here saves us any minute description of this parasitic animal. The true pimple mite was found by Henle and Gustav Simon, in 1842, almost simultaneously, and independently of each

Fig. a.

other. They are found generally and most abundantly in the glands of the skin which secrete the grease, either opening on the surface, or into a follicle, from which the hair springs. They are of very frequent occurrence, it even being asserted that no one is free from them, and are discovered in the sebaceous glands of the face, chin, nose, and forehead, by pressing out the contents of the gland, and adding a drop of colored oil to it on the glass slide of the microscope. They

sometimes occur singly; sometimes several, ten to twenty, are found in the contents of one follicle. When in large numbers, their presence may possibly cause an acne-like eruption. We have often smiled at the success of the advertising quacks, who pretend to treat diseases of the skin, in duping their victims, and in fact the public in general, in reference to this harmless animal. When a sebaceous follicle becomes, on the face or nose for instance, distended by its natural contents, the orifice of the follicle is filled with a soft, cheese-like substance, to which dirt and dust adheres, presenting the appearance of a little black dot on the skin, over the centre of a whitish minute protuberance. Pressing with the nails each side of this, and we can force out a small cylinder of greasy substance, the black dot being one end of it. Now from this *resembling* a maggot with a black head, it is generally supposed to be one; and the quack tells his clients that it is a worm of the skin, supporting his assertion by the statement that worms live in the skin. What the true pimple mites are, and their comparative size, you, however, now know; and, shall we say, should not be again duped.

CHAPTER III.

Our chapter is headed by a magnified drawing of the little animal we are to describe. It is about one-sixtieth to one-seventieth of an inch in length, just visible to the naked eye. By living

Fig. 4. Itch-mite. – Male.

in the skin of man it produces the disease known ns *itch.* To understand how to treat this troublesome affection intelligibly, we must first study the natural histoiy of the animal, its habits and habitats. Before doing this, however, it will be interesting and instructive to glance at the general history of this little creature, called in English the *itch-mite,* and in Latin, *sarcqptes hominis,* or *acarus scabiei.*

There is strong evidence in support of the idea that some of the diseases spoken of in the Bible as prevalent among the Jews were, in reality, due to the ravages of the itch-mite hi the skin. Probably, when mankind began to people the world, these insects began to people *them,* derived, by contagion, from the lower animals previously in existence. From a passage in Aristotle's "History of Animals," it has been supposed that the insect was known to him as the cause of *itch.* The old Arabian physicians, iu their writings, mention it quite plainly, – Avenzoar, for instance; but apparently we must come down to the twelfth century for indisputable reference to the itch-mite, in a work entitled " *Physica,"* written, curiously enough, by Saint Hildegard, the Lady Superior of the Convent on the Kuperts- Berg, near Bingeu. From that time downwards, the insect has been seen and spoken of by the medical writers of the times, as Guy de Chauliac,

Gralap, Benedictus, Paracelsus, Ambrose Par6, Scaliger, Fallopius, Joubertus, Vidius, Scheuck, Haffenreffer, Riolanus, Mouffet, and many others. These names carry us down to the early part of the seventeenth century, to Jansen's discovery of the microscope, in 1619. The knowledge of the use of the then primitive instrument soon spread, and the itch-mite was studied by it, the first rough drawing of the animal being given by Hauptmann. During this (the sevententh) century, the various writers on medical topics show more or less knowledge of this mite. We will not, however, tire our readers by quoting their names. Some of them mention the custom, which has been a common practice from that clay to this, of extracting the itch-mite from the skin by means of a needle. Although, by this time, the mite had been depicted, and its association with the itch disease recognized, yet it was not till 1687 that Dr. Bonomo, of Leghorn, and Ces- toni, an apothecary, studied our little friend in what we should now call a common-sense way, and thoroughly exploded the old ideas, handed clown from one generation to another, that the itch-disease was due to *thickened bile, drying of the blood, irritating salts, melancholic juices,* and special fermentation, – the presence of the itch- mite, when admitted, being accounted for by equivocal generation. These observers saw and described the insects quite perfectly, found their eggs, and discovered the females laying them, and came to the conclusion that the itch-disease, or *scabies,* arose solely from the presence of an animal which is incessantly biting the skin, and thereby causing the patient to allay the itching by scratching. They also explained the contagious character of the affection by the transference of the insects from one individual to another. Because these discoveries were true, they were denied and combated by the medical writers of those days; yet nearly one hundred and fifty years passed before any better natural history of the mite appeared. King George IT.'s physician, Dr. Richard Mead, of London, reported Bonomo and Cestoui's observations to the Royal Society, and published them in No. 283 of the "Philosophical Transactions."

We have given this little historical sketch to show how old the disease is, and how old a knowledge of its cause is also. Notwithstanding, from that time to this (1872) there has not failed to exist medical men or naturalists who deny the connection between the disease called itch and the itch-mite.' It is with medicine as everything else in the world – denial of truth excites notoriety, so desired by the many.

In view of what we have above said, it seems impossible to conceive that a correct knowledge of the itch-mite should be, since Bonomo's time, repeatedly lost in some of the great centres of medical teaching, to be again regained. In 1812, a prize was offered in Paris for the discovery of the little insect; and a certain apothecary, named Gales, gained it, by exhibiting before a medical commission the *cheese-mite.* Consequently those who searched patients with *itch* did not find *this* animal, and a prize was once more offered; and Raspail showed the cheese-mite again, and, when the judges were satisfied, proved it was such, and exposed Gales' duplicity. The cause of the itch- mite had henceforward its adherents and oppo- sers; whilst, in various parts of the world, the lowest classes understood it, and the methods of its destruction; for instance, the old women in Corsica, who picked them out with needles. Renucci, a native of the island, probably familiar with these old ladies' occupation, finally, in 1834, taught the Parisian medical world how to find the itch-mite ; and, from that time to this, the insect and its ravages have been more thoroughly and scientifically studied, and the literature of the subject grown up into quite a dermatological library. In 1846, Dr. C. Eichstedt, of Greifs- wald, and Prof. Kramer, of Kiel, independently discovered the male mite. We who, nowadays, have treated the itch-disease, and studied the natural history of the itch-mite, naturally feel as if we knew pretty much all about it; yet, so late as 1844, Prof. Hebra, of Vienna, gave the German physicians a knowledge of a uev and terrible phase of this insect's habits and habitats, iu what is known as tho Norwegian scabies, the first recorded case having occurred in that country. And so it probably will always be in the ever- advancing science of medicine, the present generation smiling at the errors and ignorance of tho preceding one. But when a truth, like the one mentioned of Hebra's, is discovered, then others are rapidly and constantly being found to confirm it. Other cases were soon reported by observers in Germany.

We suppose, by this time, our readers want to know a little more about the insect itself, and perhaps have had hardly patience to read down so far as to learn about the strange-looking animal heading our article. At present we include the itch-mite in the special class of *acarina,* and if our readers want to know more about the other members of this class, as the sugar-mite, the cheese-mite, etc., we would refer them to an article in the September number of the "American Naturalist," for 1869, by our friend A. S. Packard, Jr., who gives numerous and beautiful illustrations, accompanied by pleasantly told descriptions. What we here say will fill up this chapter for the *acarus sco. biei,* or *sar- coptes homini,* or itch-mite. The animal is tortoise- shaped. The head . distinct from the trunk, with four pair of jaws. Eight legs, four in front and four behind. The larva has but six legs. Beside the legs are long bristles. The male differs from the female in appearance, as to the bell-shaped suckers on the ends of the legs, and also is not so large. This insect has, besides man, been found in the skin of the horse, lion, llama, ape, Neapolitau and Egyptian sheep, and the ferret. It has been thought, also, that the mites found in many other animals are the same as man's irritating companion, their growth being favored or retarded by their place of development, thus accounting for the apparent differences in shape and size. The itch-mite lives in the skin, in little passages dug by itself, or, sometimes, just beneath the epidermis or scarf-skin. These burrows the animal makes extend into the deeper layers of the epidermis, down to and into the true skin, or *rete mucosum,* as it is called. The acarus moults three times, not, however, specially changing iu form. The eggs are oval in shape, quite large for the size of the animal, and may be laid by the female to the number of fifty. We give here three drawings, to show how the animal gets into the skin to form the burrows, now called " acariau furrows" by dermatologists.

In *Fig.* 5 the mite has got down beneath the epidermis. In *Fig.* 6 it has commenced digging the burrow longitudinally, and the place (/) where it was iu *Fig.* 5 has, by the gradual growth of the cells, come up nearer to the surface of the skin. In *Fig. 1,* the point (f) has thus come up to thesurface, whilst the mite has gone along further with its burrow. An animal, when it gets on to the skin, crawls till it finds a suitable soft place, when it tips up on its fore-legs, and commences to work its way in. The female, as it progresses, lays its eggs behind her in the burrow, and when

SHjpliNftR

Fig. 5.

Fig. 6.

Fig. 7.

exhausted, dies. These eggs will be seen, in a regular row behind the female, in the burrow, under the microscope with one hundred multiplying power. It is not settled how long it takes the eggs to hatch – from seventy hours to six *or*seven days. Probably onc egg is laid every day. Now, it must be remembered that the skin is constantly wearing off, and as constantly renewed by new growth from beneath; hence, as will be seen by these illustrations, the eggs hatching in the furrow will come to the surface in time for the animal to escape from its shell when fully formed. These canals which the female acari burrow, have generally a serpentine form, and are from a twelfth to a quarter of an inch in length. They show on the surface of the skin a whitish dotted appearance, the dots corresponding to the eggs – the female, as seen in the cuts, being at the *blind end of the burrow.* Ignorance or forgetftilncss of this fact has been the cause of the itch-mite escaping detection. There will be a little pimple or vesicle on the skin over where the mite went in; and, as we see from these figures, the animal is not *there,* but off at some distance deeper in the skin; hence, if we open the little vesicle, or cut it out, the insect escapes us. The old women in Corsica, and other parts of the world, knew better, and with a needle dug out the acarus from the end of the burrow. A surer way of obtaining it, and the whole burrow, is to clip this off with afine pair of curved scissors, commencing at the blind end, where the mite lies buried. Of course a little experience is required to do this successfully. Then, if we place this little lamiua of epidermis on the microscope-slide, and a covering- glass over it, but without fluid, we shall most likely find the female acarus and the eggs she has laid behind her. A magnifying power of sixty to one hundred times is quite sufficient.

After this animal had been proved to be the sole cause of the disease called *itch,* medical men thought it was always necessary to find the mite, to be sure that their patient had the itch. From the history above given, and cxplanations just made, we can see how natural it was that they should so often fail in this, and therefore conclude that their patient was not the victim of this animal parasite; consequently he was not properly treated, and did not get well – *he continued to itch.* Hence, to account for this, and cover up ignorance, was invented the "Jackson Itch," the "Seven- years' Itch," and, lately, the "Army Itch." We conclude the first did not derive its name from our former President, but was only popular during his reign. The second was ingenious ; for if apatient was told he had tho " Seven-years' Itch," he naturally concluded that he could not get rid of it in less than that number of years, which gave *time for treatment.* As time goes on, soap and water, and personal cleanliness, become more popular, hence the itch-mite has become less and less common. In the old New England days it was the pest of the village-school, the town poor- house, and the city jail. During the rebellion, the great armies, on the march and in the field, of course had no opportunities for personal cleanliness, so as to prevent the contagion of the itch- disease, therefore it spread with great rapidity by contact, and the effects of the mite's presence in the skin would also be severe. The various army surgeons had not been accustomed to any such cases; they searched in vain for the insect, and, repeatedly failing to discover it, finally concluded there must be an itch-disease not due to the itch- mite, and called it the "Army Itch." These cases often were furloughed, and, in the cities at home, came under the care of those who, from special study of cutaneous diseases, were more familiar with the means of obtaining the parasite, as wehave above described, when search for it always revealed the true cause.

This mite, in burrowing into the skin, produces intense itching, and sometimes a vesicular eruption on the surface; but this is all. The intense itching, however, causes those infested to scratch themselves incessantly, night and day; and they consequently tear and lacerate the skin in every direction. The mite, as we have said, needs a delicate part of the skin to dig into – between the fingers, for instance – and here the peculiar looking burrows are first sought for. The portion of the skin of the whole body particularly ravaged by this unpleasant parasite are so definite, that those familiar with cutaneous diseases can, at a glance, say whether the patient has the *itch.* It must be remembered that several other diseases of the skin cause as bad itching as the itch-mite; but the special portions of the general integument are, however, so marked to the-practised eye, that we no longer feel any need of finding a mite in its burrow to establish our diagnosis and treatment. In fact, we might spend a long time in fruitless hunt, when the trouble has lasted some time, or treatment has Veen attempted.

We seem, perhaps, very precise and prosy in all this; but, during and since the war, so much scabies has been diffused through our country, that many family physicians are called upon to treat what they have never before seen, and their want of immediate success should not tell against them. We only desire the community and physicians to understand that the Jackson Itch, the Seven-years' Itch, and the Army Itch, all are due to the presence in the skin of one and the same animal, namely, the *acarus scabiei,* or *sarcoptes hominis,* the itch-mite depicted at the commencement of this article.'

How now, filially, can we get rid of our minute, insinuating, and irritating friends? They lie stored away beneath the hard layer of the scarf- skin ; this, therefore, must be removed, in order to expose them; then something fatal to them, but not hurtful to the skin, must be brought in contact with them, and finally the excoriations and eruptions caused by the constant scratching must be properly treated. The severity of these latter symptoms depend, of course, on the length of time the person has been affected; that is to say, upon the number of itch-mites which are committing ravages upon him, and partly on the degree of the sensibility of the skin. As long as the person lives, the mite will flourish on him, till it is destroyed by proper methods. In the illustrations marked 1, 2, 3, the mite, as is seen, is quite deep in the scarf-skin; our first effort towards treatment must therefore be to soften and break down or rub off this epidermis. Every one is familiar with the effect of the long-continued application of warm water and soap to the skin, how it swells up the scarf-skin, softens it, and renders it easily scraped or rubbed off. Therefore a person with this highly unpleasant trouble, must first thoroughly soak himself in hot water, and rub all parts of the body which are the abodes of the mites with the strongest soft soap. This will be half an hour's work. The more delicate the skin, the shorter time required. Next, the common sulphur ointment must be rubbed thoroughly over the body. This touches and is fatal to the itch-mite, already exposed in whole or part by the burrows Ieing broken down by the soft soap and hot water. If it does not produce too much irritation, the ointment may be left on over-night, and removed by a hot bath in the, morning. With delicate

skin, sulphur soap can be used instead of sulphur ointment. If one such application as described does not suffice, it must be repeated. All the patent and popular medicines advertised lately, on account of the itch being so widely spread through the country, are pretty sure to depend for their success on the presence of sulphur, the smell of which is hid, more or less, by other ingredients. There are many other substances used by physicians to destroy this parasite. The above- described method will be sure to succeed if *thoroughly carried out,* as of course a few mites left will soon multiply and again annoy the patient. Those who are out of the reach of medicines and hot baths, may often succeed in getting rid of their minute friends, by bearing in mind the general laws of treatment; namely, that the hard scarf-skiu must be softened and broken down, and afterwards, whatever kills the acari, and does not hurt the skin, be applied. Necessity will be the mother of invention.

Nothing is more difficult, or, in fact, dangerous, than to give medical directions to be followed by the community. We would most strongly advise any one suffering from the ravages of this littlepest ta. apply to a physician, and let him conduct the treatment. Those who make a specialty of cutaneous medicine, fortunately, nowadays, have a large "choice of substances and methods of application, which can be adapted to the social condition, the degree of cutaneous sensibility, and the age and sex of the patients applying to them. This is of more importance than would at first sight appear. It must be remembered that the skin is torn and lacerated by the victim's scratching, from which we have an *artificial* inflammation of the surface, to be always taken into consideration in our method of treatment. A thick-skinned laborer needs very different applications from a delicate child, or feeble woman. We therefore again caution against self-treatment.

A single word in regard to the clothing : All underclothes should be washed thoroughly. Outside garments, contrary to the generally-received idea, do not need anything done for them. In the great hospital at Vienna, fifteen hundred cases are treated yearly, and no attempt at disinfecting the clothing is found necessary. The *mite lives in the skin.* It will therefore be seen that contagion comes from personal intercourse, particularly fromhand to hand. The most high-bred, refined, and cleanly, are not exempt. Although thus highly contagious, from the mite being passed from one to another, yet students of medicine in 'contact with it rarely get the itch; and the writer has examined and handled hundreds of cases with impunity. '. VEGETABLE PARASITES

OF THE HUMAN SKIN.

CHAPTER I.

We have given an account of some of the most common of the animal parasites which live on and in the human skin. We now propose to explain the *vegetable parasites* which succeed in growing on and in the skin and its appendages – the hairs and nails. They all belong to the class of cryptogams and order fungi, like the common moulds, seen to spring up and cover everything where warmth, moisture, and a quiet resting-place give opportunity for development. Whether they all are the same, or different species, and whether variety in soil and locality influences the form of their development, we leave for botanists hereafter to decide. It is enough for us to know that there are microscopic vegetable organisms which gp

minate in the scarf-skin of the human body, in the nails, in the little follicles from which the hairs grow, and in the root and shaft of the hair itself; and that their presence produces partial destruction or total loss of the hair or nails, and on the skin certain morbid appearances which have been classified among cutaneous diseases.

We shall confine ourselves to those which thus give rise to diseases of the skin, for there are many more vegetable growths that infest the mucous membrane and internal portions of the body. A knowledge of the presence of these vegetable organisms in certain cutaneous affections, and their being the cause of them, does not date back beyond 1840, when the microscope had commenced to reach a degree of development which rendered its use constant not only in anatomy, but also in clinical medicine. From that time to the present, scientific physicians and surgeons have steadily and constantly been sweeping the fields of their microscopes as the astronomers have swept the starry field with their telescopes, and thus from the efforts and studies of a large number of trained, intelligent, and laborious observers, the atoms of light in the heavens, and the atoms of animal and vegetable life on and iu our planet and its inhabitants, have revealed new worlds of existence to us.

What, now, are these microscopic germs which plant themselves and grow on and in our skin and its appendages ? The elements of which they are composed may be divided into three morphological formations : 1. *Spores* seen under the microscope as round or oblong cells with definite outline ; on these cells, in certain positions, is seen a brownish spot. 2. */Sporidia,* or strings of spores, looking like a rosary. 3. *Thallus fibres,* as they are called – that is, long, generally pretty straight, fibres, with double parallel outlines.

Figure 8 represents these several elements and their mode of development, which is as follows : First, a long thallus fibre increases in length, then we see contractions at several different points, giving it the appearance of a rosary, and finally by further contraction the separate spores are set free. Variety in the relative size and number of these separate elements constitutes, most probably, the various differences in the appearances seen in the cutaneous diseases which are caused by their presence. These several affections we shall describe in a future chapter, and confine ourselves in thisto explaining how and why vegetable organisms plant themselves, and grow on and in our skin and appendages.

In the first place, where do these microscopic

Fig. 8.

Showing the mode of reproduction of the

achorion. – Bennett.

spores or seeds of fungi come from? The world is full of them. They are present in all vegetable mould, and are carried everywhere by the air and Avater. The dust from our window-panes will reveal them under the microscope. The air we breathe contains them. It is with the greatestdifficulty that fungous mould can be *prevented* from germinating: for instance, in or on vegetable and animal substances. Every one knows how soon dampness produces mould. Now the vegetable parasites of the skin are, as we said, one or several species of fungi. So constant is the presence of spores in nature, that it has really become more difficult to explain why more do not germinate on our bodies than why any do. A certain and steady degree of warmth and moisture are requisite for the development of vegetable life. Besides this is needed rest and quiet of the seed, that it may take in its nourishment from the surrounding medium. Your inkstand will have no mould on it if it is in daily use. The same with your jars of preserves and pickles. A well-raked garden-path has no weeds, as also a well-tilled field. The reason why the vegetable spores do not germinate more often on the living body is, that the body's growth and *constant change of tissue,* throwing off of old to be replaced by new, interferes with their opportunity. Warmth and moisture are present, but the third element requisite to development is wanting; namely, a quiet resting-place. Hence we readily see that the more we use soap andwater to macerate and wash off the effete scarf-skin from our bodies, the less liable will the skin and its appendages, be to afford a suitable soil for the germination of the vegetable parasites. Medical experience shows this most perfectly. The cutaneous diseases due to the presence of vegetable growths are more frequent amongst the lowest classes, where dirt and lack of cleanliness prevail. But dirty persons in the upper classes are equally liable to be infested; immunity being in direct ratio to the use of soap and water. We have no need to pause here to discuss the point whether people at all ages offer a better field for the germination of vegetable spores when their bodily health is *reduced.* It is at present enough for us to know that these parasites will flourish on the most healthy person, greatly assisted, of course, by lack of personal cleanliness, because then the seeds of the fungus have all the conditions requisite for their development. In disease, one condition is to be remembered as favoring the opportunity for growth of the vegetable parasites : it is, that then the healthy renewal of tissue is either much retarded, or perhaps wholly ceases. Hence spores have a better chance to develop. Bodily cleanliness, also, during disease, is much less readily carried out, and we frequently have also the additional needed element of moisture in the fluid natural and morbid products of the skin.

How, now, do these microscopic spores get into the epithelium or scarf-skin, the nails, or into the hair-follicles, and the hair itself? The spores, from their extreme tenuity, penetrate themselves quite deeply into the cracks and fissures of the epidermis and hair, and more rapidly and still deeper when the filaments are formed. These push, sometimes merely mechanically, into readily formed cavities of the body, as in the follicles of the hair, or by elevation of the epithelium. Organic action, however, soon taking place, the hard spore presses on the soft tissue and causes resorp- tion, thus enabling the spores, filaments, and mycelium to penetrate the tissues of the body. This is only the process of germinating we see exciting such great force everywhere in nature, enabling the vegetable seed to break through its hard husk, and the young plant to push its roots into the firm soil. The penetration, therefore, of these spores into the tissues of the body, as in the case of the skin and its appendages, the hair andnails, is simply mechanical, and as readily explained as the migration of any other foreign bodies from one place in the body to another. The vegetable growth pushes aside the animal tissue. Pressure always produces absorption in the animal organism ; hence the spores, in penetrating and pushing deeper into the underlying tissue, cause atrophy of the fibres of the skin in those places. The cells containing the fat disappear, as a section of the skin will show, and a cavity is formed which is thinner at the spot where the growing parasite has fixed itself. We have, therefore, now seen where these vegetable spores come from, they being on every substance the skin conies in contact with, even the air, in which they float; and we have also seen how they penetrate the special tissues we are considering. Let us study, now, the effect of their presence and growth in these tissues.

The mere presence of the vegetable parasite in the epidermis is not of itself an injury, since it produces only slight thickening and some discoloration, with a branny condition of the surface. Unfortunately, however, itching is also caused, sometimes quite excessive, rendering the consequent scratching not only disagreeable, but posi- tively injurious. The effect of the parasites in the shaft of the hair and the hair-follicles is much more deleterious, so far as the life and growth of the hairs are concerned; for these latter may in consequence either drop out entirely, or become brittle, dry, and easily broken and rubbed off, those remaining being lighter in color, and not so strong and healthy. Absolute loss of hair from the whole surface of the cutaneous envelope may be caused by vegetable parasites, or the entire scalp rendered as smooth and free of them as a billiard-ball. Of course this must not be confounded with baldness, the result of natural or premature loss of the hair. Further than this, the presence of vegetable growth in the epidermis or hair-follicle produces an eruption of a peculiar character, simulating some natural cutaneous diseases, and causing, also, itching and consequent scratching. The nails, when infested, become brittle, dry, thickened, and crumbling. Moreover, masses of vegetable growth may lie half imbedded in the skin, which, producing loss of the hair, and being of a yellowish color, finally give the cutaneous surface a most revolting appearance, as well as simulating the products of true disease of the skin. It will be seen, therefore, that it is not only extremely inter- esting, but absolutely necessary for the physician to be thoroughly acquainted with the natural history of these vegetable parasites, so that he may be able to detect them when on the skin, or its appendages, the hair andt nails. He must also be acquainted with all their phases of development, and the appearances their presence produces, and thus be able to distinguish the effects they cause from similar ones, the result of, so to speak, true diseases. Fortunately the more extended use of the microscope by medical practitioners places this recognition more and more in their power. It is our object here, however, to let the *laity* know of their existence, and the consequences of their continued growth on the surface of our bodies.

These vegetable spores are microscopic objects, varying in size, being some thousanths of an inch. As we said, their smallness enables them to penetrate every natural cavity, such as the folds in the skin; and they are carried everywhere by the wind where dust can get. Their form is generally oval or spherical. They are very firm, so as to bescarcely crushed between the glass slides of the microscrope. Before they are thrown off they are not so firm, but more elastic and pliant. They do not lose their power of germinating by drying, except under a heat of 150 Fahrenheit. Being less dense than water, they float upon it, and are by that means also spread for and wide. They are nearly colorless – gray, brown, or yellowish when possessing any color. When in numbers,

they give a gritty feel, and mouldy taste and smell. They are not much affected by chemical agents. Tincture of iodine gives them a dark, yellowish-brown look, like other purely nitrogenous substances. When their cellulose walls are not colored blue by the action of the iodine, their nitrogenous contents become brown. On treating them with hydrochloric or nitric acid, or hot sulphuric acid, before adding tincture of iodine, the nitrogenous part coagulates, contracts, separates from the sides of the spores, and remains, forming irregular masses in the centre. On applying, afterwards, tincture of iodine to these parts, they become brown, and the cellulose walls greenish – the complementary color of the blue of the cellulose and the brown of the tincture of iodine.

The structure of the spores is very simple. All present a cell without a nucleus, unless the brown or yellowish spot on them can be considered as such. The cellulose walls are thin, but firm and resisting.

If, now, the reader has had the patience to come so far with us, he has learned that there are minute microscopic seeds of fungi scattered broadcast in the earth, water, and air, and that they can insinuate themselves into the skin and its appendages, the nails and hair. When they have thus planted themselves and germinated, they prevent the hair's proper growth and condition, discolor the skin, gather in tubercular masses upon it, cause peculiar eruptions, and are accompanied by sometimes excessive itching. All this simulates other cutaneous affections of a non-parasitic origin.

We will grant that except the loss of hair, and occasional loathsome appearances produced by the presence of these vegetable parasites, they are not to be feared or regarded with any special horror, certainly not with the extreme disgust the animal parasites involuntarily create. Why, then, is it so necessary for physicians to be familiar with theparasitic cutaneous diseases, and why also should the community understand something about them and their cause, the fungus? Our answer is simply that these cutaneous affections are *highly contagious,* by the transportation of the spores from one person to another. Every one who has had any experience in boarding-schools, day-schools, children's hospitals, etc., knows how, like wildfire, "ringworm," or "scald head," will spread among the inmates and attendants, and how difficult it is to eradicate these when once started, even with the best attention and persevering labor. It is well known, also, how a barber's shop, whose soaps and brushes are invested with vegetable spores, will spread amongst the customers a parasitic disease, which, together with some others not parasitic, gets the popular name of " barber's-itch." Some of the vegetable parasitic diseases are more contagious than others. It would also seem as if these affections were at times almost epidemic, yet we know they arise from contagion, or individual contact.

There is still another method by which the human race becomes infested: namely, from the lower animals, and these pass the parasites from one to another. Thus the following has been observed : a rat or mouse gets a vegetable fungus growing upon its skin and hair; this is communicated to the cat, which catches and plays with the animal; the child handling the cat becomes thereby affected, and finally the parents or nurse, from the infant. The peculiar contagious character of parasitic disease is, as we have said, best shown by children's schools, foundling hospitals, and the like institutions.

Finally, we hear some one ask how do any of us escape the planting, germination, and ravages of these vegetable parasites, since, when present, they are so contagious and so readily transplanted, and moreover are so innumerable in earth, air and water. It is in truth difficult to answer this, otherwise than as we have above: namely, that, like all other seeds, few find a suitable place to develop; *i. e.,* quiet, warmth, and moisture *together.* Moreover, the continual throwing off of effete material from the surface of the skin must rid us of thousands of spores which are ready to germinate. The most potent means of prevention, however, is the continual brushing, combing, and shampooing the hair, and of scrubbing the

body with plenty of soap and water. Dirt and uncleanliness are the inheritance of poverty; hence it is that among the lowest classes most parasitic diseases are found; that they are not, however, confined to them, our own experience, as that of other dermatologists, amply confirms, for we have seen enough even where cleanliness ought to be next to godliness.

CHAPTER II.

We have explained what the vegetable parasites were, where they come from, and how they penetrate and develop in the human skin and its appendages, the hair and nails. Now we will endeavor to explain more particularly the appearances on the general cutaneous envelope of the body which are produced by the presence and growth of these fungi or moulds, and also to teach our readers how, if possible, to recognize their existence, and the safest and best means of prevention and cure. This is, however, by no means an easy task, and we cannot hope to succeed so well as we did in our books on the eye, and the methods of restoring or preserving sight. The reason is, the difficulty of describing a cutaneous affection so that even those familiar with it can recognize a given case. It is, however, quite necessary that the community – the laity, as the profession call them – should have some general

idea of the vegetable parasitic growths, and the morbid or unnatural appearances they produce on the surface of our bodies. Perhaps the best plan will be to take up in turn each' disease, as there are not many, describe what it looks like, what it simulates, what its consequences are, and what can be done for cure by its unfortunate possessor, or that possessor's parents or attendants; in other words, to give a medical history, as little technical as possible, and as clearly and concisely expressed as the subject will allow of.

It must be remembered that these vegetable parasitic diseases we are about to describe, are not new affections recently appearing in the world, but are probably as old as man himself. Vegetable moulds existed before man's advent on our globe ; and when he appeared, they attacked and developed on his skin, as on that of other animals. As far back as any medical writings extend, we can trace the descriptions of diseases which we now readily place in the list of those due to the presence of a vegetable mould. It was not till about 1842, that the physician's inseparable companion, the microscope, brought to light the cause of these several cutaneous troubles, and showedus the spores, and their method of germinating on our bodies. The various fungous diseases had been, by one dermatologist after another, classed with this or that set of idiopathic diseases, according to their general resemblance. When, as years went by, and in one after another of them the vegetable parasite was discovered by the new field of inquiry being more carefully studied by many busy observers, we naturally soon arrived at better methods of treatment, and having learned the cause, soon found means of removing it, in these before so intractable complaints. The success of treatment, and the novelty of discovery, brought the vegetable parasitic diseases very prominently forward, not only amongst the profession, but also the laity, who soon learned where to apply for relief, induced by the success witnessed in other's cases. Thus some idea of these affections has spread abroad in the community, here in America, during the last ten years especially. This has given capital opportunity for travelling and advertising quacks to placard the streets, and their temporary offices, with startling and fearful pictures of these diseases, to impress the pocket and brain of their credulouscustomers. It is very true that there are enough medical men who do not advertise, and yet are arrant quacks; but it is still truer that all those who do, in any form, are sure to be impostors, who live and grow rich by fleecing the credulous. *Scald-head, honeycomb ringworm,* or, in technical language, *favus,* is the first of the parasitic cutaneous diseases we will attempt to describe. It depends on the presence of a vegetable formation, called *achorion Schonleini,* from Prof. Shonlein, who discovered the fungus. This fungus consists of numerous little oval or rounded bodies, which are the spores or sporules we described in a previous number; they are about one three-thousandth of an inch in diameter. Besides these, there are numerous tubes, varying in diameter; their subdivision forming the spores, as seen in the figure accompanying the previous article on this subject. Favus attacks three separate structures of the skin: namely, the openings of the little follicles from which the hair grows, the epidermis or scarf- skin, and the nails. The hair follicles are the most frequent seat of the disease, and it is most common on the scalp. When the fungus starts to grow, little yellow specks are seen scattered here

and there; which, under the magnifying-glass, prove to be minute rounded, bright-yellow crusts, depressed in the centre, and having one or more hairs passing up through them. These minute yellow crusts gradually and steadily increase in size, till they are about one-fourth of an inch in diameter, and then the edge is elevated above the surface of the skin. It can now be raised from its bed, and, if done with care, a circular depression is seen, corresponding to the convex lower surface of the crust; this soon fills up, the subcutaneous tissue having been compressed. A new favus cup, however, shortly makes its appearance again, unless proper means are taken to prevent it. These masses of the fungus may be scattered separately, or if increasing greatly in number, they become thickly set together, touching and encroaching on each other, thus forming irregular yellowish tubercular masses, rising considerably above the skin, in which the hairs are tangled. For other characteristic symptoms, we have itching, a change in the appearance of the hairs, and a peculiar odor of the crusts. The itching generally attracts attention first, inducing the person to scratch the affected part, and thereby produce

propagation of the affection from the scalp to other parts of the body. The hairs lose their gloss, become dull and dry, and assume a grayish or reddish color. They break more readily than natural, are often twisted or split longitudinally, and pull out more easily. When this vegetable mould has grown a long time on the scalp, the hair follicles are destroyed, and the hairs fall out, producing permanent and irremediable baldness. The sebaceous follicles, which secrete the natural and necessary oil or fat of the skin, are also destroyed, so that the parts affected become dry, and like parchment to the feel. The odor is quite characteristic, resembling that of mice; *i. e.,* a sort of mouldy smell.

The presence of the parasite, and the consequent itching and scratching, produce a certain amount of eruption and rash over the parts affected ; the neighboring glands may also swell up, and form lumps under the skin. The dirt which predisposed to favus, of course predisposes to the presence of the animal parasite which inhabits the scalp, and which we have already described. This increases the itching, and complicates the whole course of the disease. They are, however, much more

readily gotten rid of than the vegetable parasite. Favus may cover the whole scalp, and destroy all the hair. The person, by scratching, carries off some of the favus mould, and transplants it on other portions of the body. Hence, when of long standing, we are pretty sure to see patches of favus masses on different portions of the body. The vegetable matter also gets, by scratching, beneath the nail, where it takes root and germinates, as there it finds all the requisite elements for development; namely, a steady degree of warmth, moisture, and a quiet resting-place. After the spores have remained for some time, and commenced to germinate beneath the nail, the latter becomes thickened over the affected part, while the color changes, becoming gradually more and more yellow, from the favus mould shining through. As the fungus grows and increases, it gradually presses on the nail, causing further changes, the longitudinal striae become very evident, and fissures are formed. By degrees, as the pressure on the subjacent nail continues, it becomes thinner and thinner, until a perforation occurs, and then a favus cup makes its appearance externally, more or less deformed, however, owing to

the pressure previously exercised upon it from above.

In an excessive case of favus of the scalp or body, the appearances are so marked, that any one who has ever seen a case, or a good portrait of one, would be in no doubt as to the nature of the affection. But there are many other diseases of the skin, some of the appearances of which so simulate the various stages of favus, that we can hardly recommend any one, unless forced to by being away from medical advice, to attempt treatment except under the advice of a physician; not, however, an advertising quack dermatologist. The only treatment we can with safety recommend, is to soften the favus crusts in some oily substance, in order to remove them, keep up for weeks a steady daily epilation, or pulling out of the hairs, around and over the affected part, and rubbing in a solution of two grains of corrosive sublimate to an ounce of water. That this latter medicine taken internally is a deadly poison, we believe every one now knows. It does no harm externally, and serves to destroy the spores and prevent their germination. The epilation of the hairs is a difficult work, as they are very brittleand readily broken off, instead of pulled out. There is, of course, considerable risk of contagion, especially of the nails, for the operator. Favus, fortunately, is not a common disease, and is found naturally amongst the lowest classes, where misery, and its accompaniment, dirt, give a large planting field to these spores, floating in the air and water, and on nearly every substance with which the skin comes in contact. During disease, this fungus, *achorion Schonleini,* does not flourish well.

Ringworm of the head and body is the next parasitic disease we will describe. Its technical name is *herpes tonsurans,* and it is due to the presence of a fungus called *trichophyton tonsurans,* showing under the microscope the spores and sporular tubes we have above described, in the root and shaft of the hair. The first symptoms of the growth of the parasite is itching, followed by a generally vesicular eruption, taking a circular form. The hairs, where the affection exists, become dry and dull, losing their lustre, and grayish or reddish, according to the color of the person's hair; *i. e.,* light or dark. They are also twisted and very brittle, breaking off a little way above the skin, and looking as if the hair had been cut short, like a tonsure. With the continuance of the itching, the skin swells somewhat, and looks of a darker color; the fungus also appears on the hairs and surface of the skin. Finally, the hair follicles are inflamed, and the tissue around, and the matter then formed, tends to destroy the fungus itself. Thus more or less baldness is produced on the scalp, and on the body where the , hair is not so strong, and the integument different; this disease forms reddish-looking scaly rings, familiar to all as ringworm. Of course the symptoms and appearances will vary according as the disease is on the scalp or body. All sorts of remedies are popular amongst the various classes of the community. Epilation, and the application of a parasiticide, as above described for favus, are the two quickest and best methods of treatment. The success of the popular remedies is entirely due to their irritating the skin, and thus making it throw off more quickly the diseased hairs and surrounding scarf-skin.

Alopecia areata is our next disease to be noticed. It is due to the presence of a fungus called *micro- sporon Audouini,* mostly the spores above described, infiltrated, so to speak, through the hair, rendering it so brittle as to break off close to the skin. The disease has no popular same. It produces bald spots, when the hair is as cleanly removed as by the very closest shaving, the skin not showing any other signs of the disease. At first there is some slight itching, and the hairs soon commence to fall out. This may extend to every hair upon the body. Generally, however, it is confined to the head, and when occurring in a young person, gives their scalp, as smooth as a billiard-ball, a truly extraordinary appearance. When it has lasted some time, the skin becomes slightly puffy and parchment-like. It is not, apparently, so contagious as the affections previously spoken of. A patch of scalp quite destitute of hair is an important matter, especially when below where any head-gear will cover it, particularly for young ladies. When the whole scalp is clear, and the eyebrows gone, then it assumes still more importance ; for, no matter what the deceptions of fashion may be, we believe young ladies like to have *some* real hair of their own. The ravages of this parasite are hard to repair. Often the hair ceases to grow again, or only in spots ; treatmentmust be energetic, and properly conducted. Epi- lation of all the hairs surrounding a spot, steadily pursued, and the application of some remedy to kill the spores, are the means employed. Stimulation of the skin afterwards, even to repeated blistering, may induce the hair to grow again.

Barber's itch is the name which has been given by the community to the next disease to be described : *sycosis,* or *mentagra,* is its technical name. It, however, must be remembered that this name of barber's itch would also naturally be applied to ringworm on the bearded face, or, in fact, to any itching eruption of the face. Pliny described the disease perfectly, just as it raged in old Rome under the Emperor Tiberius Claudius Caesar. It was passed from one to another of the male population by their practice of kissing whenever they met. The fungus found is principally the. spores of *microsporon mentagrophytes,* which infests the hairs and hair follicles. These latter swell up into hard lumps under the skin. The surface looks red, swollen, itches, and the hairs fall out or are readily removed by the slightest pull. Pustules are formed where the diseased follicles are, and the whole bearded part of the face presents a most loathsome appearance, such as to induce the unfortunate person to submit to almost any treatment – even that of cauterizing with hot iron, employed in old Home. Nowadays the microscope has shown us the cause of the trouble, and nature points to the cure by the dropping out of the diseased hairs. Epilation, the application of a parasiticide and cleanliness, will very rapidly get rid of the disease. Ignorance of this, or ignorance of just how this should be done, the all- important point, allows many unfortunate men, not of the lower classes, to go about, a nuisance to themselves and their surroundings, from the really loathsome appearance of a part or the whole of the face. Proper treatment is very efficacious and successful.

Ohloasma, Liver Spots, are the popular names given to the last of the parasitic diseases of the skin we are to speak of, although in reality this cutaneous affection, as we shall see, has nothing whatever to do with true chloasma, or with the changed color of the skin accompanying organic or functional troubles of the liver. It is simply because this parasitic disease resembles the others in appearance, that the popular names have beenapplied to it. It is sufficient to state here that chloasma, liver spots, and the 3'ellowish or brownish discoloration of the skin, are entirely due to irregularly distributed or increased amount of the *pigment* of the skin, which, according as it is present in greater or less quantity, causes the difference of color , in the various races of mankind. The parasitic affection we are speaking of, also renders the *surface of* the skin of a more or less dark brown color; hence the laity, and, we must add, only too many physicians, confound them. The technical name of the affection is *pityriasis versicolor,* although it has nothing to do with ordinary pityriasis, the name having been given to it from its varying color, and long before its cause was discovered by Dr. Eichstadt in 1846. This cause is the presence in the scarf-skin of a fungus called *microsporon furfur*, a vegetable growth consisting of oval or rounded spores, of considerable size, and usually collected into large clusters like bunches of grapes.

Besides these Ave have under the microscope the jointed and branching tubes. The spores and tubes are also found on and in the hairs, but not to such an extent as in ringworm of the head or body.

The affection is generally seen on the trunk of the body, more rarely in the extremities, although sometimes covering the whole surface of the skin, with perhaps the exception of the head. The portions of the body covered by the clothing are most often affected. We see spots no larger than the head of a pin, up to patches several inches in diameter, and of irregular outline. These are light brown or yellowish, hardly differing from the normal skin between, or darker brown up to almost black. The larger patches are made up by the gradually spreading and coalescing of the commencing fine spots. The affected surface will be found less smooth than healthy skin, and a fine disquamation going on. The scarf-skin can be more readily scratched up, and when placed under the microscope we see the vegetable parasite amongst the epithelial scales. The presence of this mould causes itching, varying greatly in amount, hardly annoying to some persons, and to others positively unbearable. It naturally is most likely to be found amongst those classes in the community where a flannel shirt is only removed when a new one is purchased ; yet of all the parasitic affections of the skin, this is the onewhich we have most often seen in the highest and wealthiest classes. It is contagious, though not so much so, apparently, as some of the other vegetable parasites. We have seen that it does not especially affect the hairs, is principally confined to the scarf-skin, and is nothing more or less than a weed among the epithelial cells.

The proper treatment is so simple and so efficacious, that we sometimes lose our patience, when we find those applying to us have undergone all sorts of useless treatment *internally,* which is of no more service than dosing a river to kill the weeds in the meadows watered by it. We have only to macerate off the epidermis, and by the application of a parasiticide prevent the germination of the spores until they are finally entirely gotten rid of. Soaking in hot water, and rubbing with strong soft soap, will remove the scarf-skin affected , and the application afterwards of a solution of two grains of corrosive sublimate in an ounce of water is all that is needed to, in a few days, cure an uncomfortable and often suspicious-looking affection, which, without proper treatment, will flourish on the skin for a lifetime. The confounding this parasitic disease with the pigment changeof color of troubles of the liver or other organs, which the laity naturally enough do, but which physicians, at least, never should, gives plenty of opportunity for the sale of patent quack medicines, beauty washes, *et cetera,* and helps support the newspapers by the advertisements of travelling charlatans.

We trust now that our readers have, from these chapters on the vegetable parasites of the human skin, derived some idea of what the parasites themselves are, the appearances they produce on the cutaneous envelope and its appendages, the hair and nails, and the means to in some measure get rid of them, or at any rate avoid their planting themselves and growing on the surface of the body. They cannot also but be struck with the excellent opportunity ignorance offers to quackery in reference to these affections. Remember, an ounce of preventive is worth a pound of cure, and that preventive is simply plenty of soap, and lots of hot water.

FALSE PARASITES
OF THE HUMAN BODY.

Omitting those articulated animals which only wound men when they are irritated, or do not live at all upon its juices, we here give Dr. Kuchen- meister's Report on the False Parasites of the Human Body. These are : –

1. The scorpions. The common European scorpion has six eyes, and can only produce local phenomena, which are said to disappear by treatment with oils or ammonia, and in which, perhaps, collodion would prove useful. It is supposed that the effects increase with the age of the animal, and with more southern climates. The eight-eyed Indian species is said to be much more dangerous. Only local phenomena can be laid to the charge of the twelve-eyed species in Algiers.

2. The true house spiders. Their bite scarcelyinflicts a worse wound than that of a flea. However, some of the larger southern spiders may be more dangerous. Treatment with cold applications (cold earth or collodion) is sufficient. It may also be mentioned that a hysterical patient of Lopez pushed spiders under her eyelids, in order that the surgeon might remove these parasites.

3. The hunting spiders. To this class belongs the celebrated *Lycosa tarantula,* first referred to by Ferrante. Many are inclined to regard the tarantula dance, which was said to occur after the bite, as a sort *of chorea.* It appears to me that in this case too little reference has been made to the following circumstance: it may probably happen that in particular cases the bite of the tarantula may produce violent local irritation, and that perhaps it was observed accidentally by the people that violent dancing, and keeping up the perspiration in bed, quickly healed these local symptoms. To excite a desire of dancing in those who were bitten, and thus to obtain a perspiration, it is well-known that two melodies were played – the Tarantula arid the Pastorale. Subsequently this circumstance was confused or forgotten, and in courseof years it came to pass that as soon as any one was bitten by a tarantula, they played to him, and he was obliged to dance. Hence it might easily happen that people were unable to imagine a tarantula bite without its being followed by music, and, in consequence, by dancing. Thus the bite and the remedy came to be so mixed up together, that the people, and with them Ferrante, could no longer distinguish between the two. The bite is a product of the animal, the dancing a product of the music, as we may every day see in the ballrooms.

4. The bees, and humble-bees, wasps, and hornets.

5. The ants. Of course we need not here speak in detail of the caterpillars, toads, and snakes, which may accidentally wound and poison men with their bite ; nor of the lizards, if any of them are really venomous. They would not be mentioned here at all, if the popular belief had not regarded some of the last-mentioned animals, as well as salamanders, frogs, and tadpoles, certain caterpillars, centipedes, beetles, etc., as actual parasites of man, and supposed that these animals, nay, even some species of fishes, such as the eels, could carry on a parasitic existence in the interior of the human intestine. Unfortunately medical men have givep their assistance to this nonsense ; and I myself have seen one allowing himself to be fooled by a patient with an eel, and another with a frog. With such follies there are only two ways of dealing – jest and scientific experiment. The former has been done, and many, perhaps, are acquainted with the satirical tale in which a medical man in recent times has castigated a fool of this kind, who chattered about the presence of living frogs in the body of a patient, in the same style as Dr. S'. C. II. Windier *(swindler)* once derided the infusoriait theory

of the process of fermentation. But such remedies are not thorough-going, and cannot effect a fundamental cure. For the cure of these follies we are indebted to Berthold, of Littingen, and I here reproduce literally his conclusions:

1 All observations on living amphibia having remained long in the human body, and acting as the cause of long illnesses in it, are false.

2. Eggs of amphibia, when swallowed, very soon lose their power of development in the stomach. (Dr. Kretschmar, of Stolpen, informed meas an analogous case, that trout often devour fertilized trouts' eggs at the spawning time, but that these eggs, when again taken out of the stomachs of the trout, and put uninjured into fresh water, do not become developed.)

3. It is, however, possible that amphibia may get into the human subject by intentional or accidental swallowing.

4. Such animals may be again evacuated either in a living or asphyxied state, when vomiting takes place soon after they are swallowed.

5. If this vomiting only takes place at a later period, the animals thrown up are dead; if no vomiting takes place, the animals are more or less digested, and we find either their epidermis or bones, or nothing at all of them, in the faeces.

6. The only and true reason why the amphibia cannot permanently live in the human body, is the moist heat of at least eighty degrees Fah., which no species of amphibia (frogs of all kinds, frogs' spawn, the tadpoles of frogs and toads, salamanders, tritons and their spawn, lizards, and slow- worms, were employed in the experiments) can resist from two to four hours.

The method of experiment was as follows:Berthold put the animals just mentioned in vessels with water and air, which were kept from two to four hours at the temperature of the stomach, eighty degrees Fah.

The ordinary caterpillars also belong here ; they soon died, even at a low temperature, in water. They can get into the stomach with salad, or as far as concerns the smooth sixteen-footed caterpillar of *Afflossa pinguinalis,* which lives in old fat or butter, and is therefore frequently found in the kitchen and cellar with fat articles of food. This caterpillar was found by Rolander and Linne in the faeces or vomitings, and regarded by the latter as very dangerous in the human intestine. If they are soon thrown up, they are either still alive, or retain their form ; but if this takes place later, they must bear more or less distinct traces of digestion about them. In the faeces they hardly can be found again, or only in cases of very imperfect digestion, and with violent diarrhoea to drive them very rapidly through the intestines. The same applies to the *Gordius aquaticus,* which, however, from the hardness of its epidermis, may, perhaps, long resist, if not death, at least digestion. It might probably reach the stomach by the use of worm-eaten fruit.

In southern countries, leeches *(Ho&mopis vorax)* are readily swallowed with water, and these are said to be able to live some time in the human body, causing violent internal hemorrhages. This is mentioned by Larrey, and it was also experienced at the siege of Mahon.

Lastly, it may be stated, that hairs, fibres, and undigested flesh, passed with the faeces, have been described as parasites of man. The careful practitioner will be easily able to avoid mistakes.

The hair of the processionary caterpillar *(Hom- byxprocessionea),* whichforms on oaks a bag-shaped cocoon often as large as a man's head, is very dangerous to man. Nicolai's observations and researches have proved that the caterpillar usually appears during the middle of May, at first to the number of from ten to twelve, on the bark of the oak, from whence it wanders to the first buds and twigs of the oak. Each single caterpillar is from the fourth to the third of an inch in length, and of the color of the bark of the oak.

They have long, stiff, black and white hairs or bristles, and a black stripe on the back. Thislittle band of from ten to twelve caterpillars (probably relatives J keep together on a twig, and eat during night and day] They grow rapidly, learn to move more quickly, upwards of one hundred and more uniting, and forming a wandering colony, in order to attack larger branches. They wander thus from twig to twig, casting their skin for the first time towards the end of May, by rubbing against the uneven bark of the oak. They are now of from one-third to one-fourth of an inch long, of a gray color, distinctly showing twelve segments, and on the top of each segment a black shield, with very short, velvet-like hair, of a peculiar lustre. The large hairs are ranged in from two to three bunches on each segment, having lower down on their sides eight spiracles, and eight pairs of legs.

During the time of the casting oft' of the skin, the gray caterpillar becomes yellowish-brown, lustreless, stronger, but lazier. The caterpillars mostly gather where a branch withers, and attach themselves so firmly by spinning a cocoon, that caterpillar and bark seem one. The cocoon is thin and transparent, and attached to its inner part is the cast skin. These caterpillars have quitethe appearance of the former, and begin their wanderings afresh – a caterpillar leading each troop, having attached to its tail other caterpillars, and so on. They grow now very large, and collect together, at the end of June or the beginning of July, in increasing numbers. The caterpillars, placing themselves side by side, or one above the other, cast their skin a second time, and wander again, leaving threads behind on the path of their emigration. They are now excessively voracious, and deposit largely the matter which is so obnoxious to men and animals. Being now more than one inch-in length, and very strong, they are seen to make long journeys, annexing all smaller troops which they meet on their way. They gather at last on the trunk of a thick tree, placing themselves side by side to the extent of a man's hand, and then one above another, in three or four rows, after which some of the larger caterpillars are seen to creep from underneath, and spin all round the heap. The spinners are relieved by others at regular periods, and from six to eight caterpillars may be seen on the cocoon which is usually fastened to the sunny side of the trees, rarely to the stormy and northern side, at a considerable height, close to the twigs, and where a twig or branch is decaying. A hole is left in the cocoon for the passing in and out of the caterpillars, which is always guarded by several large caterpillars. These guards allow . only larger caterpillars to pass, preventing all smaller ones which may happen to follow from entering, and appointing for their use a separate place close to the nest, from whence they are led by a larger caterpillar on new excursions, to young leaves, the leader returning to its nest. The larger caterpillars deposit faeces in the nest, which, falling among the threads of the cocoon, render the latter more opaque, and more capable of resisting external influences. This closing up happens usually at the end of July or beginning of August. Each caterpillar prepares for itself a separate case or cocoon inside the large cocoon, which is of a gray-yellow color, and silk- like appearance. The single cocoons of the caterpillars resemble, in the method of their spinning, that of *Bombyx mori;* they are, however, more oval, smaller, and very rich in the yellow, powdery substance, of which we shall have to speak. The cocoons are formed in one night. The butterfly escapes towards the end of August, by softeningthe threads of its cocoon with its saliva, and thus dissolves them. It copulates, lays eggs, and dies. Many of the chrysalides in the cocoons were destroyed by white, worm-like, hairless parasites.

The inhabitants of Westphalia, in Germany, are well acquainted with the important and dangerous diseases and sufferings which are caused by these caterpillars, both in men and animals. It is very doubtful whether the noxious substance which acts like a poison, creating redness, itching, and burning of the external and inflammation of the internal parts, and causing even death, consists of the long hairs of the caterpillar. According to some writers, the nest or cocoon is to be looked upon as the cause of these disorders; whilst others say that they are . caused by an acrid noxious juice which the caterpillar is thought to seorete when it creeps over the surface of the skin. Nicolai convinced himself of the impossibility of the latter cause, for he observed itching pustules on his forearms, which were covered with clothing, though the caterpillar had never come near them. On one occasion, when attempting to attach to a board a large caterpillar by means of pins, and for this purpose piercing its black back shield, he saw onthe edge of the shield a reddish-yellow, fine, dust- like, saffron-colored powder proceed from the shield, without the latter being altered in the least. The interior of this spot showed no especial organ nor opening. Later observations, however, ar, e said to have discovered underneath these reddish spots two large warts, which almost touch one' another, and which are especially noticed when the caterpillar casts its skin, and has become deprived of its hair. The same dust was found by Nicolai in the nests and cocoons in the parts which surround the chrysalis. The caterpillar also exuded this substance on being touched with a knife on the black shields. On coming into contact with the moist skin, it caused, after eight hours, red, itching pustules, but produced no effect when

brought into contact with the dry or oiled skin.

The dust loses its peculiar power by being preserved in spirits of wine. Eatzeburg observed that feeding the caterpillars shut up in a gUss, and the necessary repeated opening of the glass, were sufficient to cause inflammation. Lameil, Physician to the Lunatic Asylum at Chareuton, observed, after the lapse of ten years even, on opening a glass which contained a piece of a cocoon,

similar *effects.* The microscope shows the dust to consist of very fine, straight, spiry, minute hairs, beset with barbs. They are exceedingly light, swim on water, and are sometimes carried away by the wind, flying about for some time in the forest. The dust is carried on to objects and into the air by the creeping of the caterpillar on a damp place, by touching it, by moving through the air, and by the falling of drops of rain on the bark. This dust seems, however, only to be formed after the second and last casting of the skin of the caterpillar. In places where the caterpillar is of frequent occurrence, the animals which come into the forests are attacked by various diseases: sheep, by inflammation of the eyes and violent coughing ; cows and goats, by the same symptoms, with internal inflammations and ulcers all over the skin, the violent itching of which, makes the animals restless, and drives them almost to madness; horses more especially suffer from it. The diseases of the eye caused by it are : Blenorrhoea of the conjunctiva, dimness of vision, and perforation of the eye. People become exposed to this poison by staying in a forest, by sleeping, working, or taking a ride, playing, cutting down wood even inwinter-time, by gathering fruit, as strawberries, which grow under the oak-trees, by collecting grass, litter, or the fallen leaves of forests. The diseases which follow are violent inflammation of the eye, erythema of the eyelids, blenorrho3a, coughing, inflammation of the throat and the lungs, violent itching and scalding eruptions of the skin (nettle-rash), and general fever. The question is, whether the above-described dust – which is found, according to Nicolai, more particularly on the edges of the black shields of each segment lining the shields with a brownish-red and delicate border, and which is velvet-like, very fine, lustrous, and soft, and which can be loosened and shaken away at the caterpillar's pleasure – be merely a mechanical, or also, at the same time, a chemical irritant; opinion differs somewhat.

Treatment and Prophylaxis. – The destruction of the caterpillars by burning and singeing them by means of wisps of straw, or by sweeping them off the trunks of the trees and crushing them on the ground, is always dangerous to the operator, since the dust is dispersed in the air. Obstacles to their migration, such as coal-tar, tarred paper, and digging trenches round the trees, are of noavail, as the caterpillar simply goes round them, and crosses even small brooks. I think it would be best to discover the nests, and wrap them up with rags soaked in oil, and then to cut away the branch, and to burn or bury it. It would be well, however, to destroy the insect in the chrysalis state towards the end of July or middle of August, before the butterfly creeps out, in order to restrict its propagation, or to hunt up and annihilate the latest brood which exists before the second casting of the skin, without the dangerous dust. It would, therefore, be necessary to search from the beginning of May to the beginning of June, for the wandering troops. The collector of nests and caterpillars will do well to use a blunt hoe, to wear gloves, and to oil the skin. There are generally only one or two nests in each tree. The caterpillar has but few enemies in the animal kingdom, of which I may mention the ichneumon. Birds seem to be afraid of it. Precautions ought to be taken to prevent persons entering infected forests by means of notices, by the digging of ditches, etc. The pasturing of animals in such forests, and the gathering of fodder and litter, should be forbidden. The gathering of fruits of

or lu.

have bee

and milk,

and lungs ai

gistic treatrq

allay and rest

. when there is .

whole, a quick au

Popular supersti from the appearance grations from west t to northern countries